# CONTENTS

# CHAPTER 1

## A History of Breakfast

Let's talk about breakfast! Have you ever been curious as to what "breakfast" actually means? Ever wonder how the ritual of eating first thing in the morning became so ingrained in our lives? People say it's terrible. People say it's the most important meal of the day. Others say they skip breakfast altogether (which is bullshit, but more on that later) and go straight to lunch. Some have breakfast for dinner. What are the rules? Why the hell are there rules? Why do people put so much bad shit in coffee to start their day? Why do people start their day with an incredibly sugary soda or energy drink that can put them in a diabetic coma just by looking at the damn thing?! When it comes down to it, the act of breaking your fast sets up the entirety of your day. Don't you want to make sure you do that right?

It's important to know where you've been before you move on to where you want to go. All journeys have that in common. And right now, you are here with me, Adam Von Roth elder, and I thank you for coming on this journey. We're going to move forward by breaking some preconceived notions of what breakfast means and ultimately make breakfast badass again! But before we take those steps let's look at how the idea of "the most important meal of the day" came to be with this brief history. Each culture has their version of breakfast and the morning rituals that come with it - even the fictional ones. Look at the Hobbits! In the Lord of the Rings movie they break it down with breakfast, second breakfast and elevens. That's how they started each day in the Shire. Probably had something to do with the leaf the Hobbit's smoked (pretty sure Gandalf and Frodo were enjoying a Middle-Earth version of Mary Jane – just saying.)

Back to the real world. What was ancient breakfast like for early humans? Discoveries by archeologists point to the Neolithic people (those around during the last part of the Stone Age) using cereal grains – this was after agriculture had become a regular thing in their lives. They ground the grains and made a type of porridge – this evidence suggests some of the first pancakes ever made! Remember the remains of that ancient human they found in the Italian Alps in 1991? They named him Otzi, and the contents of his last meal point to a type of pancake.

Let's flashforward to Ancient Egypt. Again, what was uncovered shows that peasants ate a daily meal in the morning consisting of beer, bread, and onions. I'm sure the beer helped with working on those pyramids. That was one hell of a job! In Ancient Greece breakfast was called akratisma. It was a spread of barley bread dipped in wine with the occasional figs and olives on the side. Ancient Romans called breakfast jentaculum (or ientaculum). Bread, cheese, olives, salad, nuts, raisins, and even leftovers from the previous night – typically meats – was the Roman way to start the day.

Time for the Middle Ages! The idea of eating right after you wake up (what we now know as breakfast) pretty much didn't exist. Crazy, right? People typically had two meals a day – what we now call lunch and dinner. The Church had some influence in that. The 13th-century Dominican priest Thomas Aquinas stated that breakfast in the morning was the sin of eating too soon – something associated with gluttony – which if you haven't seen the movie Seven is one of the seven deadly sins. Eating breakfast was permitted for the elderly, children and the working peasant. But it kind had a stigma attached to it. It became associated with something poor people did because the workers ate early (makes sense since they needed the energy to be productive.) And of course, exceptions were allowed for traveling nobility or if a king were on a religious pilgrimage.

In the 13th-century, they'd start the day with rye bread and cheese. Sometimes meat was included. And, you guessed it – beer! It was the low-alcohol content of course. By the 15th-century, meaty protein became a more prominent part of the experience, and noble men and women were getting down with the morning ritual. In the 16th-century, caffeinated beverages became a game changer and were included with breakfast making it socially acceptable for all and not just something the poor did.

From the 1500's on breakfast has changed as the world changed depending on culture, religion, and politics. It exists and has existed in one form or another in just about every corner of the globe. In Africa, they partake in available fruits, vegetables, and cereal grains. In Japan Miso soup and rice soup are common. In Austria, the croissant was born and was adopted by the French along with other items that we would call a Continental breakfast in the United States. We can thank the Netherlands for the waffle. In Canada, some argue that the "lumberjack breakfast" originated in Vancouver. Breakfast has been continuously changing and adapting from region to region.

It is important to note that the working class did change things. Those set schedules and long days created some hungry people. It started in the 1600s in Europe and was very widespread during the Industrial Revolution. Coffee and breakfast tea were a lot more prevalent too because of, you guessed it – caffeine! It helped in getting people going for the day when the day consisted of excruciating hard physical labor.

It is important to note that the working class did change things. Those set schedules and long days created some hungry people. It started in the 1600s in Europe and was very widespread during the Industrial Revolution. Coffee and breakfast tea were a lot more prevalent too because of, you guessed it – caffeine! It helped in getting people going for the day when the day consisted of excruciating hard physical labor.

When the hell did it become known as the most important meal of the day? We can thank a 1944 American marketing campaign for that one. It was for cereal and proclaimed that nutrition experts were saying that breakfast is the most important meal of the day. Waffles or Pancakes? Which is better? Another big question that divides America! And Bacon and eggs? There was a public relations guy by the name of Edward Bernays. He persuaded doctors to promote bacon and eggs as a healthy morning meal options to better those bacon sales Canned juices became prevalent in the early 20th century as well when people were all about the benefits of vitamins and minerals.

All that history of eating! Makes me feel hungry, to be honest. But that mix of events has led to where we are now. That history of cultures, regions, politics, profiteering, and attempts to determine what is healthy has created a bit of a messy mixed message. What we're going to do is scale things back a bit. We're going to take a hard look at what breakfast means and how important it is to start your day right in our modern society.

# CHAPTER 2

## What Does Breakfast Mean Now?

What images come to mind when you think of breakfast? Take your time and really think about it. Is it eggs? Maybe bacon? Donuts! Perhaps your favorite coffee with flavored creamer, sugar, whip cream, and flavored syrup comes to mind? How about them waffles? Pancakes doused in so much butter and syrup that the pancakes are lost like the city of Atlantis? How about cold cereal, bagels, Pop-Tarts? I bet a lot of those things come to mind when you associate imagery with the word breakfast.

The truth is, you've been conditioned to think of these things. You've been trained to mistake the food for the action. What do I mean by that? Breakfast is the act of eating after a period of fasting (usually when you're sleeping – sometimes extended if you're doing intermittent fasting – more on that later.) It is the choice of putting something edible in your mouth after an extended period of time after sleep. Let's be perfectly clear. Breakfast is not a f$%&ing waffle o pancake. It's not a cup of sugary coffee, a bagel, some donuts, and a chocolate croissant. It is the act of consuming sustenance after an extended period of not having eaten. It is a CHOICE.

Humans are creatures of habit that crave patterns and rituals. In today's society, we gravitate toward the easiest solution. We don't even f$&^ing realize we're carrying out bad habits most of the damn time because we're so used to them! It's the most common trap out there that people face when it comes to daily living. We will stick with the bad patterns that we DAMN WELL KNOW aren' good for us out of the simple fact that we've become so used to them. Want to know what the odds are to the average person making a healthy lifestyle change even when faced with a life or death situation? 9 to 1! The odds are 9 to 1 against you that you won't make a healthy change to your lifestyle even if faced with a life-threatening situation! That's f*#!ing crazy! So, how does this apply to breakfast?

Let's look at the modern understanding of breakfast. These days, people connect breakfast with eating first thing in the morning. It's associated with a product instead of an action. Meal options vary from region to region. Meals can be on the healthier side when the time allows for proper preparation, but in this day and age, we're always on the go busting our asses! Our time slots are filled with SOMETHING whether it be work, family, goals or even struggling to find more time to get more done. It's a fast-paced society of "get it to me now." As a result, a lot of convenience items have cropped up, and to be perfectly honest a lot of them are just a piss poor way in which to set the tone for your day.

Take cold cereals, for example. We grew up thinking this was the way to start the day. The reality is most breakfast cereals contain more sugar than your favorite desserts. Now let's talk about satiation (that good full feeling – not to be confused with the feeling of being bloated.) Cereal tends to leave you feeling hungry again within a matter of hours.

How about those classic pancakes or waffles? Don't get me wrong, they're delicious, but one of the main ingredients comes from refined flour. Then there's the typical high fructose corn syrup people use to drown those pancakes and waffles. That syrup could lead to insulin resistance; it can increase the risk of becoming obese and can push you along the path to type 2 diabetes. That's a path you don't want to travel.

How about Pop Tarts and other versions of toaster pastries? Easy, quick options, right? Don't let the "baked with real fruit" claim on the box fool you. The sugar is high and protein low. Lots of refined carbs that don't leave you full and lead to an increase in hunger. The majority of pastries will have this effect. Donuts, muffins, buttery scones, chocolate croissants, French toast and just about any other morning pastry that's out there.

How about coffee? Coffee in and of itself is a pretty good thing when appropriately applied to a diet. The actual coffee isn't the issue. It's the amount of shit put into coffee that creates the problem. When you start adding a TON of stuff the intake goes WAY the f&$k up. We're talking sugars (was that four packs?) whipped cream (overflowing from the top of the cup), chocolate (mixed in so it doesn't even look like coffee but chocolate milk), or one of the wide variety of syrups or a combination thereof. Man, that can turn into one calorically significant drink – especially if you're going for one of the super extra big sizes they offer because, you know, f&∧k appropriate serving sizes.

Why do we do this? It's a habit. How did it become a habit? We chose to do it over and over again. We got good at bad choices. As a result, we turned the action of breakfast into specific items that we tell ourselves we have to consume after we wake up.

I'm here to tell you it's time for a significant paradigm shift! We need to retake control, and that comes with choice. Saying you want to is not enough. It has to MEAN something to you. There needs to be a purpose that makes you FEEL it and pushes you to change – something visceral that you own. When you tap into that, you can turn this shit around.

It's like wearing a pair of sunglasses. The sun is in your eyes – it's hard to see. You're not sure where you're going. You get the right pair of sunglasses on, and you can suddenly see. You have a new perspective. Your view of things has shifted. Shift that perspective with me. Take a good hard look at breakfast and SEE what it has turned into.

I want you to think about how you start your day and how that day usually turns out. What would happen if you made breakfast the action that it is supposed to be? What would happen if you chose to balance what you consume after waking so that you're adequately hydrated, satiated and energized? You'd probably go out into the world feeling vibrant and ready to take on anything that comes your way! You'd make sure to earn the day!

That one little step – that minor change in perspective - is all it takes to create lasting change that benefits you and those you impact.

# CHAPTER 3

## A Nation of Dehydration

Bruce Lee said it best. *"Be formless, shapeless like water. Now you put water into a cup, it becomes the cup. You put water into a bottle, it becomes the bottle. You put water into a teapot, it becomes the teapot. Now water can flow, or it can crash. Be water, my friend."* This quote says a lot. It speaks to the importance of adaptation and being able to change your perspective - much like the paradigm shift we brought up in the previous chapter about seeing breakfast as an action and not a particular food. Now water isn't just important in the metaphorical sense, but it is paramount in the most literal sense. Water is life!

I want you to picture how water takes the shape of whatever it is placed in. It fills that item up. Think about your physical body. How much water do you put into it? Are you "full"? Overflowing (overhydration)? In a state of physical drought (dehydration)? Guess what? Most of your body is water. How much of your body is water depends on age and gender, but on average you are about 70% water. About ¾ of what physically makes you is water! Don't you think it's important to make sure we replenish what we lose?

Getting correctly hydrated should happen throughout your entire day. And if you're reading this, the odds are you're one of many people suffering from chronic dehydration – and probably don't' even realize it. Being thirsty, well, that means you're dehydrated – the body's thirst response is triggered by this. 75 percent of Americans are chronically dehydrated! 75%! That blows my f&#$ing mind! Basically, if we were to grab about 10 people off the street around

7 of them would be dehydrated. (7.5 to get technical, but that half person is probably on their way!) Diuretic (something that increases the passing of urine) drinks and lack of water has offset the body's water composition for most Americans.

There is also an area of our lives dehydration impacts that we don't really think about all that much. Sleep. The simple act of breathing while you sleep causes dehydration. If you breathe through your mouth it's even worse – so if you're prone to snoring or sleep apnea, you're getting even more dehydrated as you slumber. A study from the Henri Poincare University in Nancy, France found that people who breathe through their mouths suffer a 42% more loss of body fluids than people that breathe through their noses.

Don't forget about the environment. If it's hot where you sleep – guess what? Dehydration! Evening workout without replacing fluids? Dehydration! Throw alcohol in the mix. Say you were out drinking. Well, now you're just adding to the dehydration process since no one ever just goes out to have "one" drink – am I right? You're pouring down the diuretics with alcohol. Excessive consumption of liquid courage can take you to the land of dry mouth, excessive thirst, headaches, and regrettable texting.

Since fluid loss is inventable as you slumber wouldn't you say that rehydrating first thing when you wake up is kind of important? I would. Most of the research states that when you wake up, it's a good idea to drink around 16 oz of water. And depending on your body composition you might even want to drink more. If you skip water altogether and go for a fancy sugar filled special coffee drink, then you're not really setting your body up for success.

Various conditions allow for dehydration to take place. Some are illness related (flu, food poisoning, bowel disease) and some are based on your environment (not wearing proper clothing during a hot, humid day.) The more hydrated you are when you get sick, the better off you'll be because when it comes down to it, prevention is critical. The more regularly hydrated you are, the better your immune system works, and the better your kidneys function at getting rid of toxins in the body. Your joints are in a better place, and it pretty much improves your mood and overall daily performance.

I recommend you try to drink half your body weight in ounces of water. For example, if you weighed 180 pounds, then you'd drink 90 oz of water. And it's always important to make sure you're rehydrating post exercise. Especially if you're going very intense. And don't forget about your urine (an odd statement, I know.) The color is an important indication of how hydrated you are. It should be a light straw color. If it's very dark, you need to get that H2O asap.

Another aspect of hydration not often considered is electrolytes. What are they? An electrolyte is a mineral that exists as a charged ion in the body, and that is extremely important for how the cells in your body function. How does that impact hydration? As far as hydration goes electrolytes direct water (and nutrients) to the areas of the body where it's most needed. They also maintain optimal fluid level inside cells. ¡Muy importante!

Let's take a look at the starting lineup of electrolytes. We have sodium, potassium, chloride, calcium, magnesium, bicarbonate and phosphate. They all play significant roles in bodily function, and it's important to make sure your body is getting proper amounts. Making sure you start the day with appropriate levels of electrolytes is a surefire way to help set the stage for a kick-ass day.

Sodium controls the total amount of water in the body. It also helps regulate blood volume and maintains muscle and nerve function. Recommended sodium intake is 2.3g per day. Excess sodium in the body is known as hypernatremia. Happens when, you guessed it, you don't have enough water in the body. It's basically another way to say dehydration. When there isn't enough sodium in your body, well, that's known as hyponatremia. This electrolyte imbalance can be caused by severe diarrhea (not fun) or severe vomiting (also not fun.) Symptoms are likely to be headaches, confusion, fatigue – even hallucinations! Muscles spasms can happen, as well.

Potassium is a big player when it comes to what happens inside of your cells and plays a critical role in regulating the old ticker (your heartbeat) and muscle contractions. You need it for your nervous system and fluid balance. It aids in maintaining blood pressure and for overall cardiovascular health. 4.7 grams of potassium is the recommended daily intake. Most people fall way short of that. Proper amounts of potassium can also help maintain that muscle mass. Very important if you're inactive. Age-related sarcopenia (loss of muscle with age) is the real deal, and if you're physically inactive, you're looking at losing 3 to 5 percent each decade after the age of 30. Crazy! I don't know about you, but I'm all about building and preserving.

Chloride works closely with sodium. It helps to maintain proper balance and pressure of fluid compartments in the body. That would comprise blood, inside of cells and the fluid between cells. It helps keep good acidity levels in the body. 750 to 900 milligrams is the recommended amount.

Calcium – as most of you probably already know – is critical for the formation of bones and teeth. However, it is also a significant player in the transmission of nerve impulses, blood clotting, and muscle contractions. When your blood doesn't have enough calcium, it will be taken from your bones. This leads to osteoporosis. Recommended daily amount is around 1.5 grams.

Magnesium – its importance can't be stated enough. Magnesium handles over 300 biomechanical reactions in the human body and plays a role in the synthesis of your genetic code (DNA AND RNA.) It helps to maintain healthy nerve function, jumps in to help strengthen the immune system, keeps that old ticker (heart) stable, keeps that blood sugar level copacetic and promotes the formation of bones and teeth.  Around 4 grams per day is the recommended dosage. Amounts can vary depending on age, gender and if you're pregnant or lactating.

Bicarbonate is crucial with pH levels in the body. pH levels deal with acidity and alkalinity in the body. The amount of carbon dioxide in the body is regulated by the lungs. Most of this carbon dioxide is combined with water (See how proper hydration and electrolytes play a role?) and is then changed to carbonic acid. Those carbonic acids are then transformed into our friend bicarbonate, and this electrolyte is crucial for the pH buffer in the body. Keeps those pH levels where they need to be. Those on the alkaline diet will be more familiar with this process.

When you're working hard with an intense exercise, and you feel that lactic acid build up in your muscles the kidneys release bicarbonate (an alkaline solution) to counteract the increased acidity of the lactic acid. Without this, rapid changes in pH balance could be incredibly damaging to tissues around the central nervous system. This buffer bicarbonate creates is one of the reasons we can have safe physical adaptation and transformations. It allows our bodies to maintain homeostasis. The dosage of bicarbonate can vary depending on age and gender and if there are other conditions. The average range for most adults is 325 milligrams to 4 grams.

Lastly, we have phosphate. Phosphate trails behind calcium as the most abundant mineral in the body. Phosphate and calcium are like buddy cups in the old school movies. They work together to strengthen bones and teeth. It also plays a role in producing energy within a cell which is crucial for the repair and growth of tissue. It is also a building block of cell membranes and DNA. For a healthy adult, the recommended dosage is 700 milligrams a day.

All of that is a factor when your body is dehydrated. Dehydration is more severe than people realize. It can impair your cognitive functions messing with your memory, create more stress, cause you to lose focus, impair physical performance and mess with your mood. Not to mention it can help you get kidney stones – which is an experience I wouldn't wish upon anyone. Very painful.

If anything, remember what I'm about to tell you. This fact is probably the one you're going to want to commit to memory. You may find it hard to believe, but, if you don't drink water, you will DIE. Pretty straightforward. Depending on your immediate surroundings you can live, at most, a few days without any water. Maybe a week, and that's pushing it. So, if you're someone that hates drinking water try some of the following options to help stay hydrated.

Try some of the following food items to help with your overall hydration. Cucumbers (highest water content of any food), iceberg lettuce (the only good thing about it is the water content), celery (good for fiber and water content), radishes (There is a Japanese poem by Kobayashi Issa. "The man pulling radishes, pointed my way, with a radish." Radishes definitely point the way to hydration), tomatoes (It was labeled a vegetable for tax purposes. As Miles Kingston said, "Knowledge is knowing a tomato is a fruit. Wisdom is not putting it in a fruit salad. Philosophy is wondering if that means ketchup is a smoothie..."), cauliflower (packed with vitamins and phytonutrients and high water content), watermelon (great on a hot summer day), and broccoli (Raw broccoli helps hydrate with good water content.)

Remember, hydration is essential. Let's change this nation of dehydration to one of hydration, and let's get it started first thing when you break your fast!

# CHAPTER 4

## Do You Even Fast?

At the time of this writing, intermittent fasting is all the rage. Unfortunately, there is a shitload of misnomers out there about how it works and what it does to your body. It has also helped add to the false impression that you are actually skipping breakfast – and if you stop to think about it, that is f&^@ing impossible! You never skip your first meal of the day because it's YOUR FIRST MEAL OF THE DAMN DAY regardless of when you decide to eat it. We're going to clear some of the confusion up and get you on the right track.

What the hell is intermittent fasting anyway? It's basically where you go for periods of time where you eat and don't eat. It's a form of calorie restriction designed to help you maintain or lose weight. It is NOT starvation. I repeat it is NOT STARVATION – that's involuntarily going without food. It is also NOT eating as little as you can throughout periods of time. That is a type of forced starvation that can negatively impact your health. Even with intermittent fasting, you have to pay attention to your caloric intake.

Let's look back at the history of intermittent fasting, shall we?

The repackaged and repurposed intermittent fasting may seem like a new idea, but the truth is fasting is as old as human beings. It's ingrained in our history and is involved in just about every religion and spiritual practice around the world. It's been done for various reasons that extend beyond health.

Christians observe Lent. During this time on Ash Wednesday and Good Friday, people are fasting. In Islam, Ramadan is practiced. Fasting is practiced from dawn until sunset for 30 days. Yom Kippur is the Jewish tradition where fasting takes place for about 25 hours, usually starting the evening before and lasting until nightfall on the day of. In Hinduism, there are a variety of fasting practices depending on the deity being worshiped mixed with local belief and customs. In Buddhism, some monks and nuns eat only in the morning and fast until the next morning as their eating cycle.

The ancient Greeks believed fasting was beneficial from a medical perspective. Hippocrates of Cos (considered to be one of the fathers of modern medicine) often times prescribed fasting as a way to heal and get better. It was believed eating while sick only fed your ailment.

That said, it's important to understand that you should be in a good place emotionally and for the most part physically if you decide to bring a strategy like intermittent fasting into your life. If you have a history of eating disorders, have the potential to fall into one, or are already in a state of poor health, then, jumping into intermittent fasting should NOT be your first choice. Personally, I'm of the mindset to tell you NOT to do intermittent fasting.

WHAT?!!

Relax. Let me explain. Intermittent fasting doesn't make a difference. I repeat: no conclusive scientific evidence shows intermittent fasting being better than your average caloric restriction of a well-balanced diet. Intermittent fasting isn't going to magically make you have improved willpower. It won't suddenly change your eating habits. People fail diets because they just don't stick to the damn plan. Cutting things out might seem like a fantastic idea, but if you suck ass with self-discipline, then you're probably going to fail with intermittent fasting. Sadly, a lot of people out there turn it into an excuse to be able to binge. Guess what?
You don't get the results you're looking for that way.

What about autophagy Adam?

What about it?! It's one of the main arguments out there for IF, and God help you if you mispronounce it to someone that is heavy into IF (just saying.) I say who gives a shit?! Why do I say this? Because all the health markers and benefits of autophagy and reduced inflammation in the body happen just as well with a well-balanced diet where you aren't fasting for extended periods of time. Aside from slight improvements with insulin sensitivities, there aren't any real differences from those that do intermittent fasting and those that stick to a well-balanced and planned out diet.

For those that don't know what autophagy is, let me explain it. Autophagy is the process where your cells start to recycle the damaged and garbage parts. It's basically reusing your cellular components that aren't being used – the metabolic waste. Starvation tends to help this along, so it stands to reason that intermittent fasting would aid in this overall process. This process tends to happen better in the young. This process where metabolic waste in cells is broken down and recycled is desirable. The damaged cellular organelles are mainly taken care of and repurposed. This is important because it helps with the aging process. Do you need to fast to get these benefits?

Brace yourselves because I'm about to blow your f&#%ing minds! What if I told you that everyone in the world is already fasting on a regular basis? Madness! It's true. It's called getting a good night's sleep.

Sleeping is the body's natural fasted state. We're going for an extended period of time without eating, and the sleep is allowing our bodies to heal up and repair. Bonus! Now we go back to that word – the one I'm so picky about. Breakfast. We are literally breaking fast after we sleep. You've been a pro at it all your life and probably never even realized it! I can't express enough how important proper sleep is. You need it in your life. Workouts break the body down, well-balanced nutrition fuels it, and adequate sleep builds your body back up.

Now for those that do intermittent fasting, I'm not going to leave you hanging. I just wanted you to know where I stand, but if you're going to do it, then it needs to be done the right way. That means keeping track of your intake.

You can approach how you get your intermittent fasting done in a few ways. The
16/8 method is probably the most popular method out there. You're basically prolonging the amount of time you don't eat after you wake up to create a larger window of fasting. And let's not mince words here, when you're sleeping you are in a state of fasting. There's no ifs, ands, or buts about it. That's what happens. With IF you are extending that time period. So, a day of the 16/8 split would be 16 hours of fasting and an 8-hour window to get your daily caloric intake in.

Then you have the warrior diet approach to IF. You fast for 20 hours and eat as much as you want in that 4-hour window at dinner time. This approach has been known to work for some and be aware that this does take a lot of discipline. This shouldn't be the place to start if you're new to the process. This can also lead to that excuse to binge mentality. I implore you to keep track of your intake and make sure you're getting the proper amounts of macros that are also well-balanced.

The eat stop eat method is another way to get into that fasting state for more extended periods of time. You'll basically pick one or two days a week where you fast for 24 hours. The 5:2 method has you eating only 500 to 600 calories on two nonconsecutive days per week.

What do you do during the fasting state? Hydrate! Drink plenty of water. Don't underestimate this. We just talked about how important hydration is – especially when you're trying to set the tone for your day. Make sure to drink that H2O! You can also drink coffee straight up. And I mean straight up – don't add anything. That means no creams or sugars – none of that. Now I know there are a lot of people that enjoy having buttered coffee, but if you're genuinely looking to get that intermittent fasting going then buttered coffee shouldn't be consumed.

Here's the thing about buttered coffee. If you drink that, then you are essentially breaking your fast. A cup of buttered coffee is full of calories, and those calories get your system going. The point of IF is to be without caloric intake for a certain amount of time. Remember that it only takes as little as 50 calories to knock you out of the fasting state.

What about fasted workouts? Make sure you're getting those BCAA or branch chained amino acids in. You're working hard to attain the "I look sexy naked" physique, right? So help your body keep the gains you are working toward.

Herbal teas are also a great choice if you're not a coffee person. Also on the list of things you can drink are apple cider vinegar, a teaspoon of baking soda in water, sparkling water, and mineral water. You can even add a pinch of pink Himalayan sea salt to keep that electrolyte balance.

And even though stevia has no calories and doesn't raise insulin levels, I would still avoid it during the fasting state. The placebo like effect it has on the brain can cause the body to get knocked out of the fasted state. It is, after all, 300 times sweeter than table sugar. The mind is mighty and can trick your body so be cautious with stevia during the fasting state.

# CHAPTER 5

## Protein's Impact

We are going to break down protein so that you can absorb its impact. See what I did there? Protein is one of the big three. By big three I'm referring to the THREE macronutrients every human need in their system – the others being fats and carbohydrates (more on these guys later.) Protein helps with specific bodily functions, and we're going to delve into what that is, why it's important and what type of proteins you should be looking at having as part of your regular diet – especially when you decide to get your first meal of the day in.

Protein synthesis is huge! It is a critical process and making sure you have the right amounts of protein depending on your activity level is paramount. In a nutshell, the more active you are, the more you'll need. What is protein synthesis? This is the process where the body creates protein molecules. It involves amino acid synthesis (the production of amino acids.) There is also a process called transcription (genetic coding is taken from your DNA and made into templates known as mRNA.) This template is then ready for the next step which is called translation (this is where the amino acids are arranged according to the set coding that was taken from the mRNA. And voila! You have protein.)

Proteins are large complex molecules. Without them, most of the work done on a cellular level regarding the structure, function, and regulation of the tissues and organs of the body wouldn't be done. If they go on strike, you're screwed. Proteins are made up of smaller structures that we call amino acids. These amino acids are attached to each other in long chains. We have 22 different types of amino acids that can be combined to create a protein. It is the various sequences of the amino acids that determine the structure and function of that protein.

First up, **antibodies**. They are our line of defense against invaders. They bind to specific foreign particles like viruses and bacteria. They help protect your body. **Enzymes** are next on the list. These guys are incredible. Without enzymes, cells would be rendered useless. Enzymes take care of the thousands of chemical reactions that take place in the cells. They are also crucial to the formation of new molecules because they read the genetic information stored in your DNA. **Messengers.** Messenger proteins transmit signals to coordinate biological processes between different cells, tissues, and organs. Certain types of hormones are an excellent example of this like the growth hormone.

**Structural component**. These proteins provide structure and support for cells. If we're looking at the big picture, these guys also allow the body to move. Pretty significant, I'd say. Finally, **transport and storage**. These are the taxis of proteins. They bind and carry atoms and small molecules within the cells and throughout the entire body.

Alright, so our understanding is getting better. Let's take it one step further and look at those amino acids. What are they? Amino acids are the building blocks from which proteins are formed. There is a total of 22 amino acids (23 if you include ornithine.) I know, I know – you probably think there are only 20 of them. 20 are the standard ones. A few more joined the family. We'll break that down in a bit. Let's look at the categories of amino acids first. You have essential amino acids, nonessential amino acids, and conditional amino acids.

Let's start with the essentials, shall we? The body cannot create essential amino acids by itself. They need to be brought in by an outside source. In this roster of amino acids, we have the following: **phenylalanine**, **valine**, **threonine**, **tryptophan**, **isoleucine**, **methionine**, **leucine**, **lysine** and **histidine**. What does it mean if an amino acid is an essential one? Essential amino acids are the ones that the body cannot produce on its own. This means we need to find them in our diet to get them.

Then we have the conditional amino acids. These amino acids are categorized as conditional because depending on a person's health their body may not be able to produce them. A reasonably healthy person is able to create these amino acids. They are as follows: **arginine**, **cysteine**, **glutamine**, **glycine**, **proline**, **serine**, and **tyrosine**. **Ornithine** is also conditional, but it does not form proteins.

Finally, we have non-essential amino acids. The non-essential are the amino acids that can be formed by your body from other amino acids, glucose, and fatty acids. You don't need to get them from food. They are **alanine**, **aspartic acid**, **asparagine**, **glutamic acid**, **selenocysteine**, and **pyrrolysine**.

Regarding protein synthesis, branched-chain amino acids are where it's at. These include **leucine**, **isoleucine**, and **valine**. If you're looking to keep or gain more muscle these amino acids, more than any other, aid in protein synthesis.

How does this impact the breaking of the fast? If you have an active lifestyle protein should definitely be added to that first meal when you finally break your fast. In my opinion, we need more protein in our diets. As a matter of fact in a recent study Applied Physiology, Nutrition, and Metabolism *(Protein "requirements" beyond the RDA: implications for optimizing health. Stuart M. Phillips, Stéphanie Chevalier, Heather J. Leidy February, 2016)* goes so far as to suggest that the recommended protein intake that is promoted may be inaccurate. In fact, it seems that we may need more than previously thought. The study states the following:

"A growing body of research indicates that protein intakes well above the current Recommended Dietary Allowance help to promote healthy aging, appetite regulation, weight management, and goals aligned with athletic performance. Higher protein intakes may help prevent age-related sarcopenia, the loss of muscle mass, and strength that predisposes older adults to frailty, disability, and loss of autonomy. Higher protein diets also improve satiety and lead to greater reductions in body weight and fat mass compared with standard protein diets, and may, therefore, serve as a successful strategy to help prevent and/or treat obesity."

If you're kicking daily ass by making breakfast badass again and working your butt off to earn the day by killing it with your workout routines, then it behooves you to add more protein, especially for that first meal. It helps regulate and set those bodily functions for the day. It's also great for the brain and will help ensure you keep that muscle around for a long time.

# CHAPTER 6

## Fat's Impact

Let's chew the fat! Sorry. Couldn't help it.

Having fat in the morning along with your protein is a GREAT way to start the day. It's important to make sure we have the healthy fats, however, and we want to make sure we address some of the misconceptions that still run rampant regarding having fat in your diet. Fat has unjustly gotten a shitty reputation over the decades. When did this low-fat craze start? Why did it start?

We're going on a trip back to the 1950s. Heart disease was a HUGE problem. People were dying of heart attacks – and it was taking a toll. People didn't know how to combat it. Enter a man named Ancel Keys. Ancel was a nutritional scientist during a time when studying nutrition in depth was relatively new. Ancel had the theory that heart disease and diet were related. A "Seven Countries Studies" was conducted. This study recorded the diet and disease rates in different areas of the world. It looked at populations and individuals.

As well-intentioned as this study may have been, a controversial aspect of it lies in the fact that Ancel left out countries that did not support his theory of high-fat diets leading to heart disease. The countries left out had diets high in animal fats and showed low rates of heart disease. As they say, correlation is not causation. At the time he had sway over the powers that be. This guy was on the nutrition committee for the American Heart Association.

The study by Keys at the University of Minnesota really helped support the idea that fat was bad for your health. Other studies with the purpose of promoting this theory sprang up. *Hunger in America* was a CBS documentary that aired in 1968. The idea was to showcase how widespread malnutrition had become. There was also a publication titled *Hunger USA* which was written in response to the film. This all shined a big ass light on malnutrition. Senator George McGovern formed the United States Senate Select Committee on Nutrition and Human Needs. The intentions were good, but you know that road – the one to hell? It's f&$#ing paved with good intentions!

Combating hunger and poverty was what this committee was supposed to be about. It grew to encompass nutrition as a whole. In 1976 the very first set of dietary guidelines for Americans was created. In all fairness, the recommended substitutions for fats weren't that bad. The intent was to increase vegetable consumption along with whole grains and fruits. It was also essential to keep track of caloric intake (another message that got lost.) Politics and industries for profit got in the way. The message got muddled and misunderstood. All that came out of it for the general populace was the idea that fats are the villains and carbs are the heroes.

The food industry JUMPED on it! New formulas were being created to subtract fats because they saw those dollar signs. What did they add in its place? A HELL of a lot of sugars! Not to mention that convenience foods boomed post-WWII. Fast food chains started to grow in the 50s, TV dinners, the advent of microwaves, and the ability to preserve foods changed the consistency of what we were eating. We weren't just consuming raw natural ingredients any more boys and girls- some nasty shit started to crop up. Industrially human-made manufactured trans fats (not helping the image of fats) were being consumed and causing a LOT of f&$%ing harm. So we subtracted fat from everything – the taste wasn't the same – so let's add sugars and preservatives to up the shelf life and make it taste better! Screw healthy, it's about taste, but we'll say it's healthy anyway!

By the 1980s the fat-free diet was the healthy diet to follow. If you weren't following it, you just weren't healthy. Fat-free pretzels were good. Nuts were terrible because of fat. Carbs were the way to go. Fat-free yogurt, fat-free dairy – anything fat-free was good! This trend continued into the 90s. People ate a shit ton more refined carbs and sugars as a result. What happened? The obesity epidemic we're now facing.

Type 2 diabetes is on the rise, cardiovascular disease is still high (Things may have appeared to improve with heart disease from the 50s to now because of new medications and lifesaving technologies, but this is just treatment of symptoms. Taking a pill doesn't negate unhealthy eating habits.) and a majority of Americans are pre-diabetic.

The cost to healthcare in regards to all of these preventable ailments is staggering.  Imagine you're a boxer. Your coach tells you that you should keep your hands down. You keep losing matches because you're not guarding your face. The punches are coming in over and over again. You spend an entire career like this. Would you say there was progress with that career? Would you stick to that strategy and keep getting punched in the face because your coach said that was the only way to box and improve? F*&$! NO, you wouldn't! It's the same with the dietary fat debacle. Overall, the health of Americans has not seen improvement as a result of these changes.

One of the problems with Keys' research was how he spoke about abstract nutrients with a scientific mindset and didn't really go into how these nutrients should be eaten. Couple that with the need to reach as many people by catering to the masses, and you get a watered down message that skims over essential distinctions in favor of oversimplified generalizations that don't necessarily fit everyone. It was dumbed down to the point of being ineffective and essentially promoted the adverse effect.

Where does that leave us now? Ketogenic diets have shed light on the benefits of healthy fats and foods higher in fats. Paleo diets have also helped redefine the image of what a healthy diet can look like. Recent research along with previously unpublished studies have also contributed to debunking the many myths that became Gospel truth when it comes to fats.

There was a study, neglected for a very long time, which took place between 1968 and 1973 in Minnesota. It was conducted at a state mental hospital and nursing home and was dubbed the Minnesota Coronary Experiment. This study was looking at the effects of diet on heart health. 9423 men and women were chosen for this study. Half were given a typical American diet, and the other half were given a diet that replaced the saturated fat of the average American diet with polyunsaturated corn oil and corn oil margarine. The findings were FINALLY published in 2016. Someone put this study in the basement and forgot all about it to let it collect dust until recently discovered.  What the f&#k, right?!

Turns out the changes didn't lower mortality risks as theorized. Even though the cholesterol levels were lower, there was a greater apparent risk of mortality –

especially with seniors in the group. This study contradicts the idea that cutting back on saturated fat and having lower cholesterol protects against heart disease—there is more involved than just cutting the fat. The seniors that didn't cut back on saturated fat were better off.

Another study was published in March of 2010 in the *American Journal of Clinical Nutrition.* This study found that there was "no significant evidence" that saturated fat in the diet meant an increased risk of coronary heart disease. Many of the studies that have created the long-held belief regarding fat in diet had some significant flaws in them.

As far as breaking your fast goes, eating a meal with fat and protein will help balance fasting glucose levels. They will also support the adrenal gland and fight fatigue, help maintain proper energy and a balanced and improved mood, keep you satiated and help stop the dreaded sugar cravings. Ultimately, they will help avoid the ups and downs of blood sugar levels throughout the day.

Avocado, olives, (that includes the oil forms of both), egg yolks, grass-fed butter, coconut oil, MCT oil (more on that below), nuts and seeds, wild caught fish, animal fats and even coconut milk are good sources of healthy fats. Combine them with proteins such as grass-fed beef, free-range chicken, turkey, lamb, pork, sardines, eggs, quinoa and even soaked legumes and you have a good combo of proteins and fats to help balance your day.

MCT oil is a GREAT form of saturated fat. MCT stands for medium-chain triglycerides. (Sometimes they're also referred to as MCFAs – medium-chain fatty acids.) Medium is in the name because they only have 6-10 carbon atom (that's for the chemistry fans!) They are a great form of energy because they don't rely on other enzymes for absorption into your body. MCT oil has been known to help maintain healthy weight loss when included correctly in a diet, support a healthy gut, improve your cognitive functions, help with heart health, aid in diabetes prevention, and can help increase exercise performance.

When should you time your fat intake? This is something you should consider when you're on an intense workout regimen. Fats are one of those things you want to avoid eating pre-workout. Overeating fat before a workout can negatively impact that workout. They sit in your stomach longer, and your body is diverting energy for digestion instead of helping you power through your workout. Don't get me wrong – fat can improve your performance, but you should time it with other meals that aren't right before or after your workout. Post-workout sustenance should be protein and carb based, as with pre-workout snacks or meals. The protein and carbs post-workout help with protein synthesis and allow you to repair, build and keep the muscles you're working so hard to get.

# CHAPTER 7

## Carb's Impact

The dreaded carbs! (Shocking dramatic piano chord plays in the background!) Man oh man are carbs the "fats" of modern times or what? People are afraid of them. People don't want to touch carbs, or they end up giving in way too much to carbs creating a dietary imbalance. Cut carbs! Cut carbs! Cut carbs! – It's the mantra that's being placed in the minds of everyone these days. If you want to look good cut carbs. What if you could time and balance carbs out in your diet – still enjoy them – and even look and feel great? What if you didn't have to go to drastic lengths?

I'm going to put it out there. Carbs aren't the devil. That's right, I said it! Carbs aren't your damn enemy. Your habits are. Bad habits are what has made people get f&$%ing fat, and that's where the focus of change needs to be.

This is the thing: too much of anything can be bad! We've, unfortunately, had too much carb intake over the past several decades – and not the right kind of carbs either. Remember in the previous chapter about fats? Remember how carbs stepped in when officials were making people afraid to eat fat? Those refined carbs – that's where a lot of things went downhill. Like with anything, how much intake you have depends on several factors. Your age, level of activity, gender and whether or not there are any chronic health issues play a role.

Now carbs are the body's preferred fuel source. That satiation factor makes us crave them when we get a taste, which is why (refined carbs especially) can become so overwhelmingly addictive. They taste amazing! Keep in mind, however, that healthy carbs in appropriate amounts can and will benefit athletic performance, weight management, and your overall health. It's all about balance, right?

Carbs carry out many essential functions in that good old body of yours. They're a fuel source for a lot of the metabolic functions in the body and contribute to helping with brain function. When carbs are accessible, the body doesn't need to break down protein for fuel. This allows the protein to help build and repair that muscles you're working hard to get. (All about looking super sexy naked, right?)

Remember, carb and protein pre and post workout are a good combo. Believe it or not, carbs (remember, we're talking about the healthy ones) help to break down fat. They are used for energy during anaerobic and aerobic exercise and are required to efficiently break down fat.

Don't forget about fiber! Man do we need that to stay regular. Fiber is an essential type of carb (one that you can subtract from total net carbs per day if you keep track of such things) that helps with your digestion and cholesterol levels. You should be aiming to get about 25 to 30 grams of fiber per day from natural food (not supplements.)

Carbs can be broken down into simple and complex. Monosaccharides and disaccharides are the simple ones (they don't think about much.) Oligosaccharides and polysaccharides are the complex ones (deep into philosophy and existence – again, complex, so they have deep thoughts )

For starters let's delve into the monosaccharides. They are found in nature. Glucose, fructose, and galactose (that last one sounds like a Marvel villain) are the main ones. Glucose is probably the one you're most familiar with and happens to be the most abundant. It's pretty much a building block for most of the other carbohydrates.

The other simple carbs are disaccharides. These guys fall under the lactose, sucrose and maltose category. Lactose is found in dairy products, sucrose is basically table sugar, and maltose is malt sugar. Simple carbs are easily digested and absorbed - more so than their complex counterparts.

On to the complex. We have oligosaccharides and polysaccharides. The oligosaccharides are a chain of approximately three to ten simple sugars. Fructooligosaccharides are a form of oligosaccharides found naturally in some fruits and vegetables that can aid in relieving constipation, help improve triglyceride levels and help keep the bathroom a little fresher after you use it (basically lowers the foul-smelling aspect of digestive byproducts.)

Polysaccharides are starch, fiber, and glycogen. Different grains and vegetables produce starch. Starches take longer to digest and like fats can help keep you fuller longer. Fibers, like cellulose, are indigestible and are great at helping keep you regular with those bathroom deposits (you know what I mean.) Very important for your digestive health – something you don't want to take for granted. Glycogen is where it's at. This polysaccharide chain is made and stored in the liver and muscle and is an excellent source of energy for the human body. If you're more athletic, it's something to pay attention to, depending on your diet.

This is the thing about glycogen. About 90 grams can be stored in the liver (give or take) and about 150 grams can be stored in the muscles. That can be increased depending on how you train and what kind of diet protocol you're following. Now glycogen contains a lot of water molecules. 1 gram of glycogen is stored with 2 grams of water or $H_2O$. (This is where water weight comes in.) The problem most people run into is when they consume too many calories and pack on the carbs. That overage of caloric intake results in the glycogen stores converting to fat for long-term storage. Being stored with water makes them ready short term. When too much glycogen is in the body, and there is no way of expending that glycogen weight gain happens.

Glucose is fantastic brain fuel. And yes, you can also get it from converted protein and fat (the body is good like that.)  The liver is basically the reservoir of glucose for your body. It keeps that blood sugar flow steady. When you eat the liver will store sugar, or glucose, as glycogen for a later time. Then when you need it, the liver is ready to make things happen! When you're not eating the liver jumps into action transforming that glycogen into glucose. The process is called glycogenolysis. The liver can also get that needed glucose from harvesting those handy amino acids, waste products, and fat byproducts. This type of sugar or glucose production is known as gluconeogenesis.

But wait! There's more! Let's say that the body's glycogen store is running super low. The sugar supplies start to become reserved for the primary organs. We're talking about the brain, red blood cells and part of the kidney. To supplement alternative fuels are created from fats. If you guessed ketones, then you guessed correctly! This is the process known as ketogenesis. The liver really is a wonder. So take care of it, and it'll take care of you.

How you plan your day will determine how your intake of carbohydrates goes. There are many ways of approaching this based on how active you really are. If you're new to working out and new to making healthier choices, then I would recommend working on a balanced, nutritious diet that involves watching your overall daily intake. Figuring food out is hard enough. If it's new to you and you add exercise, and a timing element of when to eat you can easily overstress the old noggin,' and the brain will make you stop. The brain wins when you stress it out. The average person does well enough with a good balanced diet and exercise. Consistently sticking with that will lead to improved results.

If you've been working out at a higher level or have a handle on a nutritious, balanced diet, then timing carbs around your routines can potentially help increase the results you're going for. How about we go over some general guidelines?

First off, eat your veggies! Great carb. Great for fiber. Add in some legumes, beans, fruits, and you're good. Eat often and any time of day. Add them to every meal. Next in line are the starchy carbs. Don't run away from them! They can be very helpful and are best when eaten during that 3-hour window after your exercises session. We're talking your potatoes, sweet potatoes, sprouted grain pasta, yams, quinoa, oats, and long grain rice. Keep your portions under control and keep your total daily caloric intake in mind. This is where people tend to veer off the path.

Lastly, let's talk about refined sugary carbs. If possible, leave these out of the diet. I know, I know, that birthday party, wedding or some event comes up and guess what? There's a cake! Really pay attention to your portions and your caloric intake. Plan according to the rest of your caloric intake for that day. And if you have to have it, eat them rarely. I don't think I need to list examples of this considering we're bombarded by them all the damn time in advertising!

For athletic performance keep in mind that when exercise lasts longer than an hour and no carbs have been ingested, blood glucose levels begin to lower. (If you're on low carb or keto you can time your carb intake around your exercise, so you have that supply ready to go.) After 1 to 3 hours of endurance based continuous moderate-intensity training muscle glycogen stores might be zapped out. If no external source of glucose gets in the body, then the muscle and liver stores get eaten up. Here's the thing: it really doesn't f&%$ing matter how hard you train, or how mentally tough you are, your body will feel it, and it will impact your performance.

Carb loading is a sound strategy for anyone competing in or training for long-distance endurance events. We're talking marathons, triathlons or primarily any activity that typically lasts more than 90 minutes. So if you're a sprinter carb loading isn't for you. If you're serious about carb loading for optimal performance consulting a sports specific dietitian is advised.  The pros and cons of carb loading are many when you implement it in your training regimen, so best to have a trained professional guide you through the process and help tailor the right food plan for the goals you're trying to accomplish.

You also have the option of the pre-exercise snack. The goal with this is to optimize the availability of glucose in your body and provide fuel for your body to give that exercise session everything you've got. Exact timing to eat before exercise depends on the person as the digestive process can vary from person to person. Play around with it, and give yourself enough time. 1 to 2 hours before with a snack is an excellent place to start.

What about during exercise? Can you fuel up? I'd only recommend that during prolonged sessions. We're talking marathon status, or for the average person sessions that last longer than 1 hour. This can help address that problem of "hitting the wall" that a lot of long distance runners experience. If it's less than 1 hour, the body should have enough glucose to last. It is recommended that athletes consume 30 to 60 grams of carbs per hour of training.

Recovery! The best part of the exercise – when you're done with it! The goal is to replenish your glycogen stores and help facilitate that good ol' muscle repair process in the body. Carbs and protein are a great mix for post-workout recovery (they are the buddy cops of the recovery process.) The carbs replenish the stores, and the protein can focus on repairing the muscles. The amount of refueling depends on how hard you've trained.

If you're the average person getting it in within that 3-hour window works just fine – within that first hour is even better. But if you're an athlete timing might be different depending on how vigorous your training is. Typically, a range between 2 to 4:1 ratio of carbs to protein depending on your overall dietary needs/choice, and intensity/duration of the training session.

So, in a nutshell, be smart about how you use carbs. They aren't the enemy, but abusing them can lead to a lot of problems when it comes to managing your weight and being healthy overall – especially if you stick to those tastefully but oh so bad for you refined sugary carbs.

# CHAPTER 8

## Balancing Macros

There is the familiar physical form of balance we've come to know. Being on one foot, handstands, walking on an unsure surface, and a plethora of yoga and martial arts poses that can keep you busy for years. But what about balance when it comes to what we eat? What about balance when it comes to breaking fast? If we don't take care of our physical balance, we're worse off. Why wouldn't the same hold true for our dietary balance? If you want to set a proper tone for your day, then you need to start it off right, and balancing your intake is a huge part of that.

By this point, we should all have a solid understanding of what the main three macronutrients are and a good idea of what they do for the human body. I'm talking about proteins, fats, and carbohydrates. So when we decide to break our fast, how do we put this all together? Where is the proper balance?

So, let's get this out of the way first. Everyone is different regarding how they respond to food, and everyone is different regarding what they can realistically manage. There are a plethora of choices when it comes to how you want to eat throughout the day. There are some things you need to factor into your decision-making process.

One is your level of activity. How active are you? If you're more active, then you'll need to consume more food. If you enjoy doing the math, then we have equations ready to go for figuring out your daily caloric intake. There is also a timing factor that some people choose.

Remember, these are tools, not the law. You just need to find the right tool that works for your purposes. As long as you're getting the right amount of calories per day and stay consistently close to that number, then you'll start seeing some good results. Add an excellent exercise program that fits your goals and needs, and now you're really talking!

Daily caloric intake. Basically, we're looking at how much you're consuming throughout the day. As a human being, you require a certain amount of calories to maintain regular daily functions. This caloric number represents the amount of energy needed to maintain homeostasis – when the body is balanced and at rest – basically not being super active. You can go online and find a BMR calculator to do the work for you. You'd be looking up the Harris-Benedict formula. If you like doing the math yourself and checking the numbers, then the equation goes as follows.

Finding your basal metabolic rate:

For women: BMR = 655 + (4.35 x weight in pounds) + (4.7 x height in inches)–
(4.7 x age)

For men: BMR = 66 + (6.23 x weight in pounds) + (12.7 x height in inches) – (6.8 x age)

Once you have this number, you know what your set point is. You then take that number and multiply it by an activity factor.

If you are sedentary (not active): BMR x 1.2 = caloric intake for the day

If you participate in light activity (sports or exercise 1 to 3 times a week): BMR x 1.375 = caloric intake for the day

If you are moderately active (sports or exercise 3 to 5 times a week): BMR x 1.55 = caloric intake for the day

If you are very active (hard exercise 6 to 7 times a week): BMR x 1.725 = caloric intake for the day If you are extra active (tough exercising/sports – super physical job or training twice a day): BMR x 1.9 = caloric intake for the day

We can scale down the numbers even more if the equations feel like they're too much. You can keep it simple with a calorie per pound approach. This method allows you to stay focused on maintenance calories for your desired body weight. For example:

If you're looking for fat loss multiply your bodyweight by 12-13. That number will yield a ballpark number of about how many calories you should take in for fat loss.

Standard maintenance calories are where you're happy where you're at, want to keep working out, but see better results without dropping weight. Take your bodyweight and multiply it by 15-16. That will give you about how many calories per day.

Lastly, you want to gain weight. Say you have a hard time keeping that lean muscle on. Then you would take your desired bodyweight and multiply it by about 18-19. That number will be about how many calories you should take in.

Let's say you're 180 pounds and want to maintain that weight. You would take 180 pounds and multiply it by 15. 180 X 15 = 2700 calories per day.

Play around with it. Make adjustments as needed. It's not about hitting this perfect number every day. It's about being within that range – close to – consistently. That is the discipline: consistency.

Now you have your daily caloric intake. We're going to stick with the 2700 calories since we started the example with that number. We are going to take that 2700 calories and figure out the proportion of macros you need. Again, macros are your proteins, fats, and carbs (we just spent 3 chapters on each one.)

Getting a handle on your macros goes a LONG way. If you can walk into a grocery store, read that label, and know what kind of macros you are looking at you are golden when it comes to sticking within your range of calories for the day.

Percentages are up to you. It depends on what you're going for. If your diet is more keto, low carb or paleo you'll have a higher percentage of fats and a smaller percentage of carbs. If you follow a DASH diet, you'll have more healthy carbs and low fats. A Mediterranean style diet would be higher in healthy carbs, and low in protein.  There are different ways for different people depending on what they have going on healthwise. So ALWAYS stay in communication with your doctor when making these kinds of changes.

Keep in mind you'll have to play around with macronutrient percentages. This is not and never has been a one size fits all. But if you play within the right ranges, you will see the results you're looking for. We're going to use ISSA recommendations as a gauge.

Let's say that you have always been skinny and have had trouble putting on the pounds. You're looking at a starting point of 25% protein, 55% carbs, and 20% fat.

Now let's say you're more on the athletic side and have an excellent muscular frame. Your starting point would then be 30% protein, 40% carbs, and 30% fat.

Lastly, let's say you have a slower metabolic rate and a lower tolerance for carbs. That ratio will look like 35% protein, 25% carbs, and 40% fat.

Me personally, I like to keep my physique in check all year long. I need to be tiptop given my profession and my personal goals. My particular breakdown falls around the following: 40% protein, 30% carbs, and 30% fats. This is my range. I'm higher or lower on specific macros depending on more specific goals, but this guideline suites me personally. It's no secret I believe protein is SUPER essential to your health and fitness goals.

Again, it's a range. You WILL find yourself playing around with the ranges. It's inevitable, and it is something you should welcome. That's how you learn. That's how you get better at it.

We're going to use the 30:40:30: macro breakdown from above to continue the example with 2700 calories.

For Protein: 2700 X 30% (that turns into 0.3) = 810 calories. 810 is then divided by 4 (this is because there are 4 grams of protein per calories of protein) so 810/4 = 202.5 grams of protein.

For carbohydrates: 2700 X 40% (that turns into 0.4) = 1080 calories. 1080 is then divided by 4 (this is because there are 4 grams of carbs per calories of carbs) so 1080/4 = 270 grams of carbs.

For Fats: 2700 X 30% (that turns into 0.3) = 810 calories. 810 is then divided by 9 (this is because there are 9 grams of protein per calories of fat) so 810/9 = 90 grams of fat.

Do your best to keep your meals balanced with all three macros. And it doesn't matter how you break it up so long as you're getting in the ballpark of 2700 calories per day (for this example that is – your number depends on what you come up with.) You can do 6 smaller meals a day, you can have 3 meals a day with some snacks, you can do intermittent fasting and how one large meal and one smaller meal, or even break down 3 meals during the eating phase. You can also do the intermittent fasting where you have only one large meal a day. It's about what works for you and how it can fit into your lifestyle. To be honest, I'd avoid the intermittent fasting approach, but that's me.

And if numbers freak you out remember that you can use your hand to determine portion sizes. Your hand in relation to you is a good indicator of roughly how portion sizes should go.

Make a fist with your hand. The size of that first is a cup of carbohydrates (yes that includes veggies.) Now open your first and straighten your fingers revealing your palm. Your palm is a serving of protein – roughly 3 to 5 oz. Keep your hand open with fingers out. See your thumb? Your thumb size is approximately a portion of non-oil fats (butter, etcetera) and is about 1 tablespoon. Look at the back of your hand. Extend your pointer finger. The tip of that pointer finger is a serving of an oily fat. That would be about 1 teaspoon.

# CHAPTER 9

## Fuel the Brain

The brain is a marvel. It's incredible that we have brains when it comes right down to it. Our brains take care of so much shit for us, but it's equally important that we take care of the ol' noggin. That involves feeding it the proper fuels so that we ensure our brain is functioning at full capacity. Fats, carbs, and protein all play their part when it comes to maintaining a healthy brain. Here's a quick breakdown of what happens with the brain and the three macros.

To put things in perspective, it's important to understand that your brain is one extremely hungry sonuvabitch. It CRAVES nourishment. The human brain is only about 2 percent of the body's total weight, but it uses up to more than 20 percent of your daily energy intake to function. 20 percent! What we eat will impact the brain's fuel source. We're talking about how you feel, how you problem solve, how you remember, and how your brain runs all the background "programs" if you will, that allows your body to function without you consciously thinking about it.

If your brain and carbs were officially dating the description under relationship status would read: It's complicated. If you give the brain carbs, it will gobble that glucose down like it's going out of style. When that glucose loving brain starts to run out of that source things happen. Hypoglycemia (low blood sugar) being the main result. This is when you get lightheaded, your balance is off, and confusion. It's important to recognize these symptoms and some carbohydrate-rich food (the healthy stuff, remember.) Carbs are the body's preferred fuel source when it comes down to it. kicks in.

There's a difference between cutting carbs entirely and ending up in that hypoglycemic state and restricting your carbs - like if you were on a low-carb or ketogenic diet. Restricting carbs can impair brain function in the short term. Your body is resilient, however, and can adapt and find other energy sources by turning proteins into glucose through gluconeogenesis (a need driven reaction), or fats get turned into ketones as a source of energy, and the brain will gobble up the ketones.

So with carbs remember that vegetables and fruits are carbs. They're not separate from that. Half of a meal should have vegetables – the nutrient dense kind. Whole grains are what we go for, refined grains are what we stay away from.

It has been shown in various studies that over time a fat-free or low-fat diet can really impair your cognitive functions. On the flip side, a diet higher in fats has shown to improve cognitive function, especially those more on the keto end of the diet spectrum. If the keto diet is too much the Mediterranean diet is another possibility when you take time to consider what would work for you. So take in those healthy fats. They're good for the brain.

Now the body is excellent at adapting. I've mentioned it several times before. Through gluconeogenesis and ketogenesis, the body can provide ample energy to the brain with an overabundance of carbs. It takes on average, about two weeks to become keto-adapted after living a life full of carbs (usually the bad kind in the standard American diet.) Ketones created from fat help by being a neuroprotective antioxidant keeping brain cells healthy. They also aid with maintaining the aging brain so that it functions better, help improve function with neurotransmitters in the brain, and ketones help trigger BDNF (brain-derived neurotrophic factor) which helps with learning, memory and overall higher thinking.

Let's go back to our friend protein. Protein is fantastic for the brain a variety of ways. Adequate amounts of protein can help curb reward-driven eating. So you'll be less likely to go for that extra slice of pizza, eat those cookies, or indulge in those treats. When that protein reaches the small intestine, it releases CCK (cholecystokinin) which travels to the brain and acts as an appetite suppressant. Protein also helps control the hormone ghrelin. Ghrelin has been known to persuade the mind to act impulsively. When eating that translates into I can't believe I ate the entire tub of ice cream. Protein can help wrangle that hormone in and keep the brain a little steadier with the decision-making process.

Protein also raise levels of an amino acid called tyrosine – the brain booster! This amino acid prompts the brain to create norepinephrine and dopamine which are basically chemical messengers in the brain. These keep you energized, alert and allow to feel like being more active.

Overall, it comes back to balance. If you keep your diet balanced and healthy, then that will positively impact your brain functions as well. When we eat we often only consider how it affects our physical body, but our brain is a factor we shouldn't forget. And it is an essential factor. So keep that diet balanced not only for your body but so that you can achieve and unlock all the cognitive potential waiting                      to                      be                      unleashed!

# CHAPTER 10

# Badass Mentality

Why do people fail when they attempt to make a positive lifestyle change? This has been a huge question I address when working with people to improve their lives. The research out there shows us that the odds of you making a significant lifestyle change (even when you're facing a life-threatening situation – i.e., the possibility of a terminal illness), is 9 to 1 against you. 9 to 1 against you! That's how hardwired your brain is to the habits you've created over time. How do we break that? How do we beat the odds and get that life we want, that body we want, and overall the success and joy that sustains us instead of draining us?

We've discussed how we can make breakfast badass again through a balanced approach to nutrition. We've touched on how that food impacts your cognitive functions as well. It's about setting the day right, and proper nourishment for your body and mind will get you started in the right direction. Once you get started down that path, you need to work that mental strength in a way that will sustain you not only physically but emotionally and intellectually. Balance applies to the mind as well as the body. It starts with your perspective because that will dictate how your day goes.

Martha Beck said it best. "The way we do anything is the way we do everything." Those ingrained patterns work their way into just about every facet of our lives. If we start our day with a negative outlook that perspective will become the filter of how we see everything else as the day goes on. Tommy Kono, an American say practice makes permanent." Practice in and of itself isn't the key – it's practicing things well that makes the difference. And guess what? If you practice the bad habits and work on being negative with your outlook every day you're going to get pretty damn good at having that shitty perspective!

So what do we do? First, we need to find a way to hack the brain. We need to tether ourselves to something that can get us through the bombardment of negative thoughts and perspectives. That thing you need is an anchor. For me, anchors have been crucial to my development. Anchors are what keeps us grounded while the storms of life rage on – minor storms to significant storms. They help us keep the big picture in mind and allow us to move forward because those anchors are there to remind us that we're grounded, but yet are able to walk with us as we take our personal journeys.

I want you to think about what your anchors are. What are the things that keep you grounded when you can't make sense of what's happening around you? It could be family, friends, or an activity. For some it's meditation, exercise can definitely be one, and martial arts are another example. It could be reading, writing or any artistic or creative endeavor that allows you to express yourself.  It could be the teachings of a mentor or memory of a loved one that can help guide you. It can be spiritual or religious so long as it is helpful and allows you to zero in on that better version of yourself that you're trying to achieve.

Contrary to popular belief willpower runs out eventually. It doesn't last. That's why people end up hitting their breaking point if they try to force change through sheer will alone. The anchor helps with that. When things feel overwhelming you anchor, reset, refocus and allow that to create momentum. Now I've always said it's not motivation but momentum that gets you there. We can be motivated to do a million different things, but that motivation fades. We have to hone in on our goals in a way that makes it accessible to the part of ourselves that loves what we're trying to accomplish and do. The part that is fed with the little goals we achieve and perpetuates that move forward.

So when our anchor has served its purpose that anchor is aweigh (raised clear.) We're bringing it back to us, so we can stow it and take it with. A lot of nautical descriptions here, but you get my point. We can keep moving with the momentum created by the new pattern – that new pattern being the positive places we go when we need to (the anchors.) That gives us the reset we need, and we keep kicking ass and breaking down the obstacles that get in our way by either using those obstacles or riding out the storm.

My recommendation is getting that first anchor set, and that first anchor should be how you start your day. For me, I have a movement routine I do every morning that gets me primed for the challenges of the day. It gets my mind right, and I'm ready to conquer my tasks and the unexpected things that pop up. So a combination of proper nutrition and hydration when you wake up – making sure to break your fast in a way that's conducive to a positive outlook – and a morning anchor can help you set the proper tone for your day.


With the right anchors, a funny thing starts to happen. You begin to earn the day. What do I mean by this? I'm talking about E.A.R.N. the day. Education, Activity, Relationships, and Nutrition. I like to say that I live the white collar life with a blue-collar mentality. You see, anchors help you find purpose. Purpose is nurtured when you E.A.R.N. it. Whatever your calling – whatever your goals – it's important to cultivate the four pieces of E.A.R.N.

Education. What sticks with you more? When someone tells you about something or when you experience it for yourself? Probably the latter if you're like most of us. We start out getting information from others. That's normal. We're told, we then read and then we're researching on our own. It's important not to get lost with one methodology or mentality when it comes to the information you take in. Always learn from your environment, other people, and most importantly your own experiences. Explore as you educate yourself and you'll find that there is always more to learn. Make the education portion enriching. Learn something each day that will make you better. And the more knowledge you have, the better you'll be at solving problems. Solving little problems on a regular basis gives you the fortitude to tackle the big goals.

Activity is pretty self-explanatory. We need to move. The body LOVES to move! You determine just how much movement you're going to undertake. Consistently getting a little activity in every day goes a long way to remaining healthy and living a long full life. It's something that can actually help add years to your lifespan if you stick with it. So find something you enjoy doing – something you love that puts a smile on your face. It should be something you look forward to doing when you think about it, and something that gets you moving – an activity you genuinely enjoy. Combine the education aspect with activity, and you're discovering and learning while being active! It could be a detailed workout program, to walking every day, to swimming, surfing, martial arts         –         the         sky         really         is         the         limit!

Relationships. Where would we be without them? We get strength from those around us. So wouldn't you want to surround yourself with people that support you and help build you up instead of bringing you down? Staying close to family, friends and loved ones on a regular basis helps balance that emotional state. It can also give you the extra push you need to accomplish the goals you have set in your mind. Cultivate your relationships. Find positive role models and mentors. Stay in touch with those you care about and find that support. Being strong in these relationships will allow you to be strong with other more professional relationships because the confidence you need will be there. Combine this with the previous two parts of E.A.R.N. Learn with those closest to you and be active with those close to you, and you'll have a strong tribe that is ready to keep

kicking ass!


Nutrition is always key. We've spent quite a lot of time in this book talking about it. So I'll keep this brief with a few key reminders. The body you have right now is the only one you get. We don't have the technology to switch bodies at this stage of the game, so we have to treat the ones we were born with well. Nutrition provides the fuel you need to keep going not only physically but cognitively. We've touched on how food impacts the brain, mood, and emotions. Don't cheat yourself on this aspect. It really does help provide the proper balance needed to be the version of yourself you want to be, and to go out there and kick ass on the regular!


Want to live the white color life with the blue color mentality? Then E.A.R.N. it! Cultivate knowledge and experience, actively DO – being aware of your body and moving it, create lasting relationships in your personal and professional life, and lastly get that nutrition in check. Building these qualities will give you the stamina to keep your anchors strong. If you're able to keep your anchors strong, you can deal with the grind and knock down whatever obstacles are in your way. E.A.R.N.                              the                              day!

# CHAPTER 11

# Looking Sexy Naked

We have arrived! Are you ready to delve into a strategy that will help you look super sexy naked? This simple approach to balancing everything out and putting it all together will help you to get that sexy body, so you can look in the mirror and say, "Damn! I look good naked!" And who wouldn't want to look good naked, right? Now I know that's not what it's all about – we're also looking at improving our overall lifestyle and health. Sometimes that takes intrinsic goals (motivations that come from the inside) and extrinsic goals (motivations that come from the external sources – like I want to look good naked!) The external goals will lead to the internal ones. It just takes that commitment.

So, by putting together all the lessons you picked up from the previous chapters let's start with the internal. Find your anchors, get them set. Draw your inspiration and strength from them. E.A.R.N. Now restructure your narrative. How do we do that? Remember what we've talked about. Start your day right! Let's set it up with the proper balance of nutrition.

In Chapter 8 we discussed balance and breaking down the macronutrients appropriately. You figure out your caloric intake for the day by using the equations set for BMR and activity level or by multiplying your desired weight by the appropriate number range for calories per pound of bodyweight. You then break down that caloric intake number into the percentages of macros. Again, my personal range is 40% for protein, 30 percent for carbs, and 30 percent for fats.

That could be different for you depending on your goals. Refer to macronutrient percentage ranges set up in Chapter 8.

What was that? How do I start the day, you ask?

I get my coffee going and make sure I'm hydrated properly. A good cup of Café Latte from Strong Coffee Company is where I start. The fast has been broken, right? And I break my fast with a liquid to get my digestive system set properly for the day. I get my morning routine going to get moving – one of my anchors. A few hours later I get my serving of oatmeal and have my eggs. Veggies with the eggs of course – need those veggies! My day is off to a great start! I've moved and given my body what it needs to set a proper narrative for the day. My mind is sharp and focused. Hell, I even get some work done in the morning taking care of a few things right out the gate because I'm focused.

What was so great about how I started the day? I moved to get my mind right. I gave my body the nutrition it needed. I worked – even working a little bit goes a long way to reaching those goals. I allowed myself to feel. I felt how my mind connected to my body, I allowed myself to process whatever I was feeling and used it in a positive way to get my morning momentum rolling. I allowed myself to feel the enjoyment of the process from waking, to coffee, to moving, to working and to the rest of my breakfast. Move, work and feel. This will help get you the control you need at the start of the day.

Keep that balance to your nutrition throughout the day. Remember that is super important. Have veggies with all your meals. Make sure there are adequate protein and fat. Lots of water for hydration. Stay strong with the balance and work on the blunders that come from what I refer to as narrative dilemmas. Narrative dilemmas stem from the unfortunate overexaggerating that has bled into our perspectives of how we view ourselves and others. People tend to stick to their "convenient truths" that target a pain point in someone's life by solving a problem with skewed science made to fit what a person wants to hear.

This is where the faulty math comes into play.

1.) I eat all day long and need to lose weight.

2.) If I eat only half of the day, then I'll just be half of the weight!

3.) Total Weight From Eating All Day – Weight Achieved from Eating Half the

Day = PERFECT

WEIGHT GOAL! YAY! Guys, that's not how it works.

Once you have your macros figured out (again refer to Chapter 8 to obtain your exact numbers) you then delve into the something I've found to work with all of my clients. It is a straightforward rule to follow that has helped me to change the lives of countless people that have now achieved their goals.

I'm just going to assume that everyone wants to be in the best shape that they can be in and look super sexy naked. Throwing that out there. It's a place to start with goals, anyway. So you're figuring out your meals for the week. Let's say you have 21 meals per week at 3 meal per day (might be different for you depending on how you choose to break it up with when you eat.) You start by making sure that 80% of those 21 meals are clean and healthy, and the remaining 20% of those meals are the things that you use to treat yourself a bit. So approximately 17 meals are healthy, and the remaining 4 are where you allow for treats to happen.

STICK TO YOUR DAILY CALORIC INTAKE! I can't stress that enough. Don't go overboard on calories. Keep the range correct. Otherwise, this isn't going to work. There are a TON of useful apps out there. Myfitnesspal, Mynetdiary, and Nutrtionix are just a few.

Now, let's say that special day or beach time vacation is coming up. You want to change it up more if you're looking to get that nice cut, lean body with the envious abs going on. So about 6 to 8 weeks before that special day you change up the percentage. 90% of what you're eating needs to be healthy and clean, and only 10% of your daily intake is where you can make room for the treat yourself meals. Let's stick with 21 meals. That would mean 19 meals are healthy and clean (21X90%) and 2 meals per week can be allotted for the more indulgent stuff.

Let's say you are ready to go all out and you want to make it to that unicorn status. Then, my friend, you're looking at a 95/5 split. 95% of your meals are going to be healthy, and you're only allotting yourself 5% of those meals per week (again based on your total daily caloric intake) as treats. That would break down to about 20 (21X95%) clean meals a week and 1 meal where you can allow the treats to have their time.

I want to talk more about that narrative dilemma when it comes to your workout routine. When I own and operated my own gym people would regularly say things like, "Man you gotta try this workout – it f%#@ing killed me!" That always bothered. It bothered me because it doesn't give people the proper narrative. To someone that doesn't know me, how I program, and what the workout is like – it's just going to sound like someone is doing something batshit crazy that they aren't going to want to try.

The minute I started asking clients to not describe the workouts in that way was the minute that newer faces began showing up interested in trying out the classes and sessions. You see, as a people, we tend to exaggerate things. We've all done it. You and me. We take an experience and make it out to be 10 times more than what it was in either direction by playing it up or down. When it's something we might not have the motivation to do in the first place those exaggerations take center stage, and the voice inside telling us not to do it sounds pretty damn reasonable in comparison.

To find your place in that spectrum you need to find that consistency. This is where the anchors help. E.A.R.N. the workout (Education, Activity, Relationships, Nutrition.) Keep it simple to start. A lot of people tend to say that they don't have the time or can't make the time. This drives me f#$@ing bonkers! Saying you can't make time is a copout!

The ancient Roman philosopher Seneca wrote the following:

"It is not that we have a short time to live, but that we waste a lot of it. Life is long enough, and a sufficiently generous amount has been given to us for the highest achievements if it were all well invested. But when it is wasted in heedless luxury and spent on no good activity, we are forced at last, by death's final constraint to realize that it has passed away before we knew it was passing. So it is: we are not given a short life, but we make it short, and we are not ill-supplied but wasteful of it... Life is long if you know how to use it."

When I need a good kick in the ass about time and how I use it, I think of Seneca. My takeaway is this: the exaggerations about not having enough time are keeping you from achieving the body and health you are capable of. Too often we make time for the things we "believe" we need. This is based on those convenient truths. We neglect what we actually need as a result. There never seems to be enough time for anything. It all slips away, and we're left thinking we can never make it happen.

That's bullshit!

A 30-minute workout is still a 30-minute workout no matter how you slice it. We all have the same amount of time given to us. We can work it so that we give our mind, bodies, and souls the things we need to flourish. Guess what? That 30-minute workout a day is totally doable. Take a good hard look at how you're spending your time and be honest with yourself about it. How much time are you using vegging out in front of the TV watching movies or shows? How much time is spent telling yourself you'll make time for it later when you have time as you think about it? We take time to make time. That's always been the balance, but we live with a constant imbalance because we're taking time to make time for things that aren't genuinely making us better.

Don't get me wrong. We need the downtime – just like we need the meal that's not as healthy as the others. You can apply the 80/20 split for your time as well, and when things really need to get done get that ratio to 95/5.

Whatever the workout program you're attempting, whatever your goals are, you can achieve it. Start your day right by breaking fast the right way. Anchor yourself with the positive things that will nourish you. E.A.R.N. those anchors and activities as we've discussed. Start simple and let it naturally flourish, and you'll be on a path to a better version of you. It's the version that is in there waiting to get out, and it is my sincerest hope that the world gets to become well acquainted with that person.